The Health Care Decision Guide *for* Catholics

How to make faith-based choices for
medical care and life-sustaining treatment

Patricia D. Stewart

Foreword by Rev. Ronald K. Tacelli, S.J.

SWEET APPLE PRESS ✳ NORWELL, MASSACHUSETTS

The Health Care Decision Guide

for

Catholics

How to make faith-based choices for medical care and life-sustaining treatment

By Patricia D. Stewart

Published by:
SWEET APPLE PRESS
P.O. Box 770
Norwell, MA 02061

Book and Cover Design: Sue Charles, Marshfield, MA

©2007 by Patricia D. Stewart

First Printing
Printed in the United States of America
ISBN-13: 978-0-9702465-0-9

Imprimatur: Most Rev. John Mulagada, D.D.
Bishop, Diocese of Eluru, India

Dedication

For the greater glory of God
and the Roman Catholic Church

Acknowledgments

⁓

My heartfelt thanks and appreciation go the following persons, who made this book possible:

my mother, Gloria, for sharing with me her gift of faith;

the Reverend James E. Braley, the Reverend Lancelot J. Reis, and Tom Flaherty, for inspired insights and thoughtful reviews that helped shape the message of this work;

Myra Doran, for her unceasing support and prayerful encouragement;

Louise Marciano, for sparking the research behind the book;

Judith Bruce and Claire Sussek, for believing in me as only life-long friends can;

Sue Charles, for designing the cover and formatting the text;

the Reverend Ronald K. Tacelli, S.J., Ph.D., for ardently affirming the project and writing the book's Foreword;

Frank Kelly, for inestimable spiritual support and for opening all the doors necessary to the realization of this work: and

Our Blessed Mother Mary and Saints Joseph, Thomas More, and Francis de Sales, for guidance and intercessory prayers.

Contents

≈

Foreword

⁓

It was all so simple then. Those who are old enough remember what it was like to be taught about the Last Things. Heaven or Hell lay before us. Either we would make it and enjoy the presence of God and the company of the saints forever (though most of us would have to pass through the vestibule of Purgatory to get there); or we would lose everything and suffer that ultimate loss for all eternity. Those were about the only end of life issues we Catholics felt compelled to deal with. And for most us, they were more than enough.

But now medical science has changed all that. The same discoveries that have eased our pain, sustained our breathing, nourished us when we could not swallow, replaced our organs and have thus, for countless people, made the burden of life more bearable have also, at the same time, given rise to burdens of their own: hitherto undreamed-of questions, dilemmas, crises.

If you've ever dealt with the contemporary health care system on behalf of a terminally (or just seriously) ill loved one, you know exactly what I mean. Will we nourish? hydrate? resuscitate? And if not, what will we do with the body? Bury, cremate, or perhaps donate? Catholics may dimly remember something about not having to sustain life by extraordinary means. But what used to seem extraordinary seems nowadays pretty ordinary. When is it right to refuse treatment for yourself? For another? Should the notion of quality of life enter into your decision? If so, how? And what about the alleviation of pain? When is it right to use medication that will eliminate pain but also shorten life?

These questions are neither academic nor avoidable. The world we now live in demands that we face them. Some of us, in fact, have faced them already whether or not we were equipped to do so. And that's the point of this wonderful little book: to prepare us to deal as faithful Catholics with the new Last Things.

We all owe Patricia Stewart a special debt of gratitude for *The Health Care Decision Guide for Catholics*. It's subtitled *How to make faith-based choices for medical care and life-sustaining treatment*. And, like any first-rate how-to book, it's practical, clear, concise, and direct—in every sense user-friendly.

When the stakes are as high as life-or-death, a friendly, faithful guide is as much as we could pray for. In that sense, *The Health Care Decision Guide for Catholics* is literally Heaven-sent.

RONALD K. TACELLI, S.J.
BOSTON COLLEGE

Starting or Continuing Medical Treatment

A faith-based decision about whether to begin a proposed medical treatment or to continue treatment that is in progress depends upon whether the treatment is reasonable in the circumstances of each case. To determine the reasonableness of a medical treatment for yourself or someone else, start with the general decision-making standards of the Catholic Church arranged below as four questions. Carefully consider each question by answering all of its sub-parts.

When you have answered all applicable questions, a "Conclusion Box" suggests the appropriate faith-based choice derived from your answers. Then, before you reach a final decision, review the specific standards in Chapter II and follow any that apply to your case.

Deciding on Medical Treatment

Questions 1 and 2 establish the circumstances for your decision; Questions 3 and 4 address the consequences of the treatment. It is important to answer all of the questions *in the order presented.*

To help organize your thoughts, write your responses in the spaces provided.

1. WHO IS THE PATIENT?

Age:_____

Position and responsibilities in life (for example, a
father who is the sole support of a large family):

_____

_____

_____

_____

_____

_____

Physical and financial resources:_____

_____

_____

_____

_____

Psychological status and available moral support:

_____

_____

_____

_____

2. WHAT IS THE MEDICAL TREATMENT?

Name:_____

How complex or simple is it to administer? (This matters because a complicated treatment may not be reasonable.) _____

_____

_____

_____

_____

_____

_____

What is/are the risk[s]?_____

_____

_____

_____

_____

_____

_____

What is the cost?_____

_____

_____

How easy or difficult is it to obtain? (This matters because a treatment that is difficult to obtain may not be reasonable.) _____

_____

_____

_____

_____

_____

_____

_____

Is there anything unreasonable about it? _____

_____

_____

_____

_____

_____

_____

_____

_____

_____

_____

3. WHAT IS THE EXPECTED RESULT?

Given all of the circumstances identified in your answers to Questions 1 and 2, does the treatment offer a *reasonable* hope that the patient's condition will improve?

⭕ YES   ⭕ NO

CONCLUSION:

If your answer to Question 3 is "NO," the treatment *may* be refused or discontinued. Do not answer Question 4, but before making a final decision, read Chapter II and follow any standards that apply.

If your answer to Question 3 is "YES," go to question 4.

⬥❈⬦

---

4. How will the treatment affect the patient and the patient's family and community?

Will it subject the patient to extreme pain?
O YES   O NO

Will it subject the patient to danger?
O YES   O NO

Will it subject the patient to serious risk?
O YES   O NO

Will it impose excessive cost on the patient
or the patient's family?
O YES   O NO

Will it impose excessive cost on the
patient's community?
O YES   O NO

Continued ☞

CONCLUSION:

If you answered "YES" to *any* part of Question 4, the treatment *may* be refused or discontinued, but before making a final decision, review Chapter II and follow any standards that apply.

If you answered "NO" to *all* parts of Question 4, the treatment *should* be started or continued.

Health Care and Life-Sustaining Treatment In Special Circumstances

In addition to the general decision-making standards identified in Chapter I, the Catholic Church gives explicit guidance for health care and life-sustaining treatment decisions that involve issues of:

+ anatomical gifts

+ cremation

+ euthanasia

+ imminent and inevitable death

+ lack of a remedy using ordinary medical care

+ nutrition and hydration

- pain
- physician-assisted suicide
- pregnancy
- quality of life
- vegetative state

When any of these circumstances or issues exists, the guidance of the following specific standards should govern your decision.

Anatomical Gifts

The gift of the patient's body, body part(s), or tissue for purposes of organ or tissue transplantation, therapy, scientific research, or medical education may be made with the consent of the patient, or if appropriate, his or her duly authorized health care agent or representative or other person authorized by law to so consent.

Cremation

A Catholic may choose to be cremated without obtaining permission from the Church; however, this choice may not be made for reasons that are contrary to Christian teachings. The request may be verbal or written as part of the person's will or advance health care planning document.

When exceptional circumstances—such as financial hardship, limited burial space, or unsuitable geography—preclude the burial of a body, a family may decide to have an individual cremated; however, this should seldom be done against the individual's wishes.

The cremated remains of the body should be placed in a proper container (commonly an urn) and should be buried in consecrated ground, entombed, or buried at sea. They may not be scattered, distributed to survivors, kept at someone's home, or made into other objects.

Euthanasia

Euthanasia, defined as doing something or failing to do something *with the intention* of causing death for the purpose of ending suffering, is *never* an acceptable health care choice.

Imminent and Inevitable Death

When the patient's death is imminent and inevitable, treatment that will prolong the patient's life in an uncertain and burdensome state may be refused or discontinued, as long as normal comfort care—such as cleanliness, warmth, nutrition (food), and hydration (water)—continues.

Nutrition and hydration should continue, *even if provided by artificial means*, as long as doing so nourishes the patient and alleviates his or her suffering.

Lack of a remedy using ordinary medical care

When ordinary medical care cannot improve or cure the patient's condition, he or she is not required to undergo extraordinary medical treatment in the form of the most advanced medical technique if it is experimental, risky, or excessively costly. Instead, the patient may accept ordinary medical treatment with its limitations.

Alternatively, the patient may consent to receiving extraordinary medical treatment. In this case, before deciding to pursue the treatment, the decision maker should consider the following four questions *in the order presented:*

1. WHAT ARE THE *REASONABLE* WISHES OF THE PATIENT AND HIS/HER FAMILY?

_____

_____

_____

_____

_____

_____

_____

_____

_____

2. WHAT IS THE ADVICE OF DOCTORS WHO ARE EXPERT IN ADMINISTERING THE TREATMENT?

_____

_____

_____

_____

_____

_____

_____

_____

_____

3. WHAT IS THE COST OF THE TREATMENT, INCLUDING INSTRUMENTS AND PERSONNEL? ($_____) IS THIS COST EXCESSIVE GIVEN THE FORESEEABLE RESULTS?

○ YES   ○ NO

4. WILL THE TREATMENT SUBJECT THE PATIENT TO EXCESSIVE SUFFERING GIVEN THE FORESEEABLE RESULTS?

○ YES   ○ NO

CONCLUSION:

If you answered "YES" to *either* Question 3 or Question 4, the extraordinary medical treatment may be refused.

If you answered "NO" to *both* Question 3 and Question 4, the extraordinary medical treatment may be pursued. But note: it may be discontinued with the patient's consent if results are not as expected.

Nutrition and Hydration

The patient should receive nutrition and hydration (food and water), *even if provided by artificial means,* as long as doing so affords the patient nutritive benefits and alleviates his or her suffering. It is only when these objectives can no longer be achieved that nutrition and hydration may be withdrawn. See also "Imminent and Inevitable Death" and "Vegetative State."

Pain

When the patient is in pain, medicines may be used to relieve suffering.

When no other options exist, pain relief should be given even if a medication decreases the patient's consciousness and unintentionally shortens the patient's life.

Note, however, that the patient should not be rendered unconscious without a compelling reason.

Physician-assisted suicide

Assisted suicide of any kind is *never* an acceptable health care option. Thus, physician-assisted suicide, the act of voluntarily ending one's life with the assistance of a doctor or other medical professional, is *not* a permissible health care alternative.

Pregnancy

When the patient is pregnant, no treatment may be undertaken or omitted with the intent of causing the patient's death, or the death of the unborn child, for the sake of preserving one life over the other.

If the patient is dying, she should receive life-sustaining treatment if such continued treatment will benefit the unborn child.

Quality of Life

The inherent value and personal dignity of a human being never change, whatever the physical circumstances of the individual's life. This essential truth transcends any person's judgment as to the quality of another person's life. For this reason, decisions about a patient's medical care *cannot* be based on considerations of the "quality" of the patient's life.

Vegetative State

When the patient is in a vegetative state, he or she has the right to basic health care, including cleanliness, warmth, nutrition (food), hydration (water), and the prevention and treatment of conditions caused by being bedridden; he or she also has the right to beneficial rehabilitative therapy and to clinical monitoring for signs of improvement.

Nutrition and hydration must be provided, *even if by artificial means*, as long as doing so nourishes the patient and alleviates his or her suffering.

Planning for the Future

Few decisions in life are as stressful as those concerning health care or life-sustaining treatment for oneself or someone else. A little advance planning can go a long way toward reducing the anxiety and uncertainty of these choices. It can also ensure that, should you become incapacitated, medical decisions made for you will be faith-based. Here's how:

A Four-Step Plan:
Share, Select, Sign and Send

1. SHARE your beliefs about health care and life-sustaining treatment with family members, friends, health care providers, or others who may be involved with your future medical care. *TIP: Use Chapters I and II as a guide.*

Some people become uncomfortable or fearful talking about these subjects. If you encounter resistance from those around you, remind reluctant listeners that your purpose is to protect them from anxiety and confusion in the event that you become unable to make health care decisions for yourself. Point out that talking about serious health issues does not forecast their happening any more than discussing health insurance foreshadows an accident or illness. These conversations are merely sensible means of planning for the unknowable future in every life.

2. SELECT someone you trust to make health care decisions for you should you become unable to make or communicate those decisions for yourself. Then, choose someone else who will decide for you if your first choice is unable to serve. Neither person has to be a Catholic, but it is vitally important that they understand your beliefs about health care and life-sustaining treatment decisions and agree to do their best to make medical choices for you according to Catholic standards.

3. SIGN an advance health care planning document. A health care proxy (also called a health care declaration) and a health care power of attorney are legal documents that allow you to officially appoint the people you chose to make health care decisions for you in the event that you become incapacitated. These documents must be executed (signed) according to the statutory requirements of the state in which you live. If in doubt, consult an attorney about the proper procedure in your state.

When you appoint someone to act for you, you are called the "principal." The first person you appoint is called your "agent" or "attorney in fact." The second person you appoint is your "alternate" or "successor" agent and serves only if your first agent is unavailable. Some states use different titles for the people you appoint, but all of these individuals have similar powers and responsibilities. For simplicity, we will use the term "agent" in this discussion.

A health care proxy/declaration takes effect only after you have been found to be incapacitated or unable to make or communicate your own health care decisions. A health care power of attorney may take effect either when you sign it, or at a later time, depending on what you say in the document.

Your agent's authority *begins* when your document takes effect; your agent's authority *ends* when you regain decision-making capacity, revoke (cancel) the document, or at some other time that you may specify in the document.

The authority of your health care agent includes the power to decide for you whether to accept, continue, discontinue, or refuse medical treatment, including procedures that may sustain or end your life.

You can instruct your agent how to make health care decisions for you. Do this initially when you talk with your prospective agents before appointing them to represent you. *(See Step 1)*. Then, write down your instructions, either as part of your health care proxy/declaration or health care power of attorney or as a separate document, often called an advance directive for health care. Although the names of these advance health care planning instruments vary from state to state, all states permit you to include instructions based on your religious beliefs. *TIP: Contact Sweet Apple Press for a copy of the Catholic Statement of Beliefs and Decision-Making Standards. Attaching these instructions to an advance health care planning document will make it faith-based. Order by email: www.orders1@sweetapplepress.com or by U.S. mail using the Easy Order Form in the Appendix.*

4. SEND a copy of your executed document to your agent and alternate agent or your attorney in fact, as the case may be. Also, send copies to your physician and the hospital or other health care facility where you are admitted currently or are likely to be admitted if you require medical care in the future. Tell your doctor and the hospital to include the copies in your permanent medical files.

Lastly, send a duplicate original or copy of your document to the attorney most likely to be involved if a dispute arises over your future medical care. Keep your original document in a safe place, and let someone know where it can be found if needed. *TIP: Complete the card found in the Appendix, stating that you have executed a Catholic advance health care planning document. Then, place the card in your wallet for use in an emergency.*

Review

Reread your advance health care planning document periodically to be sure that it accurately reflects your wishes and that the persons whom you have appointed to represent you are your current choices. Should you desire to make changes, execute a new document. CAUTION: Do not merely write in new names on your old document as this may have the effect of cancelling the entire instrument. See "Revocation" below.

Revocation

If you change your mind, you can easily revoke (cancel) any advance health care planning document. Most states recognize acts taken by you that clearly show your intention to cancel the document, such as telling your agent or physician that you wish to revoke your proxy/declaration, crossing out or destroying the document, or executing a new one. In many states, if you appoint your spouse as your agent and later are divorced, this automatically revokes your proxy/declaration. Ask an attorney about the accepted cancellation methods in your state.

Reciprocity

Many states accept an advance health care planning document that has been executed properly according to the laws of another state. This practice is known as reciprocity.

Therefore, if you reside in more than one state, you may not need to execute separate documents for each location. An attorney can advise you about your state's reciprocity laws.

Living Wills

A living will is a document in which a person provides instructions for when to withhold life-sustaining treatment in the event that he or she is suffering from specified physical or mental infirmities, such as terminal illness, extreme pain, persistent vegetative state/coma, and other conditions in which one's "quality of life" is considered to be undesirable. *(Note: A living will does not dispose of your material possessions at the time of your death.)* Some states have other names for this type of document, such as "declaration as to medical treatment" or "advance health care directive." Whatever name is used, the document's distinguishing characteristic is an advance refusal of medical care. For simplicity, we will use the term "living will" in this discussion.

To the extent that a living will rejects life-sustaining treatment prematurely, without regard to the circumstances of the patient's life or the consequences of the treatment and motivated by "quality of life" concerns, it contradicts the Catholic standards in

Chapters I and II and, thus, is not a desirable health care planning tool.

If a living will is the only form used in your state for providing advance health care instructions, be careful to revise it to reflect Catholic teachings before you sign. *TIP: The Catholic Statement of Beliefs and Decision-Making Standards available from Sweet Apple Press can be attached to a living will to make it conform to Catholic standards. The Statement is available by U.S. mail using the order form in the Appendix or by email: www.orders1@sweetapplepress.com.*

Do-Not-Resuscitate Orders

A do-not-resuscitate order is a document in which a patient, or his or her health care agent or representative, agrees in advance to the withholding of cardiopulmonary resuscitation procedures or medications in the event of the patient's cardiac or respiratory arrest.

If the patient is capable of making his or her own health care decisions, only the patient can consent to a do-not-resuscitate order. If the patient lacks decision-making capacity, then his or her health care agent or representative may make the decision. In either case, a decision to issue a do-not-resuscitate order should be based on the same considered judgment applicable to other medical treatment decisions, as set forth in Chapters I and II, and should not be based on quality of life concerns. ✤

Appendix

Sources for Further Reading

Codex Iuris Canonici (Code of Canon Law), cans. 1176 § 3, 1184 § 2.

Committee on the Liturgy, National Conference of Catholic Bishops. Order of Christian Funerals, Appendix: Cremation. Chicago: Archdiocese of Chicago: Liturgy Training Publications, 1997, nos. 415, 417.
_____.Reflections on the Body, Cremation, and Catholic Funeral Rites. Chicago: United States Catholic Conference, 1997.

International Commission on English in the Liturgy. Order of Christian Funerals. Chicago: Liturgy Training Publications, 1989, nos. 406.1-406.4.

John Paul II, Pope. *Evangelium Vitae* (The Gospel of Life). Boston: Pauline Books & Media, 1995, ¶¶65, 66, 86.
_____. (address to the 18th International Congress of the Transplantation Society, Rome, August 2000).
_____. (address to the International Congress on Life-Sustaining Treatments and Vegetative State: Scientific Advances & Ethical Dilemmas, Rome, March 2004).
_____. "Bishops Must Stand Firm on the Side of Life, Against the Culture of Death-Encouraging Those Who Defend It" (address to United States Catholic Bishops of California, Nevada, & Hawaii, Rome, October 1998).

Pius XII, Pope. "Medical and Moral Problems in the Practice of Resuscitation" (address to an International Congress of Anesthesiologists, Rome, November 1957).
_____. "Religious and Moral Aspects of Pain Prevention in Medical Practice" (address to the Ninth National Congress of the Italian Society of the Science of Anesthetics, Rome, February 1957), 145, 147.

Sacred Congregation for the Doctrine of the Faith. "Declaration on Euthanasia." Rome: Sacred Congregation for the Doctrine of the Faith, 1980, II-IV.

United States Catholic Conference, Inc.--Libreria Editrice Vaticana. *Catechism of the Catholic Church.* New York: Doubleday, 1995, ¶¶2270, 2278, 2279, 2296, 2301.

INDEX

SWEET
APPLE
PRESS

Booksellers

Easy Order Form
on reverse side.

SWEET APPLE PRESS
EASY ORDER FORM

BY E-MAIL: www.orders1@sweetapplepress.com
OR COMPLETE AND SEND THIS FORM
BY MAIL: Sweet Apple Press, P.O. Box 770-B Norwell, MA 02061.

I wish to order:

Title	Quantity	Total
The Health Care Decision Guide For Catholics	____ @ $7.00/ea.	$_____
Catholic Statement of Beliefs and Decision-Making Standards	____ @ $10.00/ea.	$_____
	SUB-TOTAL	$_____
Sales Tax: Please add 5% for all items shipped to Massachusetts addresses		$_____
Shipping: US: $2 for each book $2 for each Catholic Statement of Beliefs		$_____
	TOTAL DUE	$_____

SWEET APPLE PRESS

Booksellers

Payment method enclosed: ❑ Check ❑ Money Order
Ship to:
Name_____
Address_____
City _____State_____Zip_____
Telephone_____
email_____

You may return any item for a full refund if not completely satisfied.

48

After you have executed your advance health care planning document, complete this card and keep it in your wallet or purse.

IN CASE OF MEDICAL EMERGENCY

_____

MY NAME

I HAVE EXECUTED A CATHOLIC ADVANCE HEALTH CARE PLANNING DOCUMENT.

Please call my health care representative,

or alternate health care representative,

identified on the reverse side of this card.

HEALTH CARE REPRESENTATIVE

TEL:_____

ALTERNATE HEALTH CARE REPRESENTATIVE

TEL:_____